THE SECRETS
OF
AYURVEDIC DETOX

By
MONICA RAMIREZ

Copyright © 2015

www.wellnesshealthhub.com

ISBN-13: 978-1517107376

ISBN-10: 1517107377

Disclaimer

The information provided in this book is designed to provide helpful information on the subjects discussed. This book is not mean to be used, nor should it be used, to diagnose or treat any medical condition. For diagnosis or treatment of any medical problem, consult your own physician. The publisher and author are not responsible for any specific health or allergy needs that may require medical supervision and are not liable for any damages or negative consequences from any treatment, action, application or preparation, to any person reading or following the information in this book. Any references included are provided for informational purposes only and do not constitute endorsement of any websites or other sources.

Please accept my gift to you, a complimentary report with great tips on how to achieve maximum results when detoxying. Click here to get your free ebook http://wellnesshealthhub.com/ayurvedic-report

Check out my other books on Amazon :

15 Minutes Daily Workout That Will Kick Your Butt Into Shape

The Complete gluten free diet

Contents

Introduction

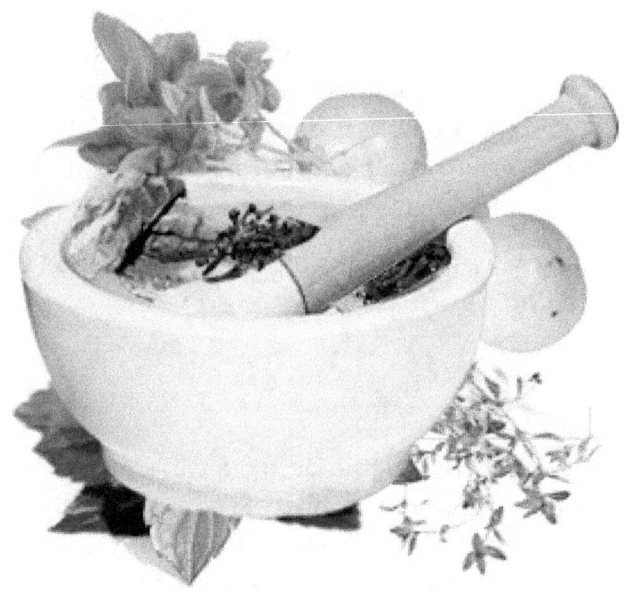

Source: newstrackindia.com

Ayurveda is an ancient medical system that began in India. Unlike most other medicines, Ayurveda is considered to be completely natural. This book is about Ayurvedic detox, and in other words, it is the cleansing of the body by removal of toxins.

Normally, toxins develop in the body during winter, and the period where the weather changes from winter to spring is actually considered the best time for Ayurvedic Detox. A normal, full fledged Ayurvedic Detox program takes 15 days of preparation. But the actual procedure will take one and a half months, that is 45 days. Overall, the Ayurvedic detox procedure will take a total of 60 days to complete. This is equal to a period of two months.

You can lead a normal life during the Ayurvedic Detox process, but you will have to follow a diet. The digestive system must perform well and should not be exerted, and at the same time, the detoxification process is carried out.

Many people try to exert themselves too much during any detox process, but that is not needed. In fact, if you exert yourselves, you will not get the complete benefit. *The Council of Maharishi Ayurveda Physicians* gives a clear, detailed information about how to carry out the detox process.

While this book will provide information from various sources, the basic do's and don't's are as follows.

Do's:

When undergoing an Ayurvedic Detox, always prefer organic food. Vegetarian food is always the best. Fruits, grains and spices are the best foods. A mixture of fresh yoghurt (curd) and water called Lassi is a good beverage that is needed for everyone. It also provides stamina. Warm lemon water is also a very good detox agent.

On the other hand, it is essential that you do not choose foods as you like. All the three *Doshas* must be pacified Consult an Ayurvedic specialist, or strictly follow the instructions given in this book. Not all recipes might taste good, but when you need detox, you need to follow these procedures.

Don't's:

These are the things that you should never do while undergoing Ayurvedic Detox. Avoid foods that do not digest easily, or cause incomplete digestion. Do not eat non organic food (anything that is packed or made artificially). Even fruits and vegetables should be organic. Heavy dairy products should be avoided, although fresh Yoghurt is allowed.

Deep fried substances, oily products, heavy desserts, too much of sugar and honey is also to be avoided during Ayurvedic Detox. You should also try to refrain from eating breads, crackers, and other type of yeasted food.

It is also good to avoid meat. Processed meat, leftovers, or any of such kind is very bad while following your detox diet. In fact, it is very good if you avoid all these for the rest of your life. Ayurvedic Detox normally involves a vegetarian diet, and we suggest you to follow that as well.

Either way, these are the things that you should not do when you are on an Ayurvedic Detox diet. All this will be explained in detail in the forthcoming pages. There are many views and ideas about Ayurvedic Detox, and in this book, you will find the combination of the best methods.

There are three phases of Ayurvedic Detox that you will have to undergo. These are known as the pre detox, detox, and post detox phases. They are also known as pre cleanse, cleanse, and post cleanse phases, so do not get confused if you come across these wordings.

While this book will contain recipes of diets that should be followed, you should also note that it is just a guide, and you will have the liberty to frame your own plan. The book will include a basic outline, and then it will include the details of the detox or cleansing stages.

There will also be diets for breakfast, lunch and dinner. It is up to the reader to form your own schedule. You can choose from the recipes and diets you like, but you will have to stick to the detox schedule and the diet very strictly.

Ayurvedic treatments also focus on the mind, rather than the body. Hence, a mental approach to the detox process is also essential. Normally, Ayurvedic Detox processes require a relaxed mind and a comfortable scenario.

Do not try to undergo this procedure if you are unwell, recently recovered from an illness, or if you are not in a good state of mind. It will be nothing more than a waste of time. You can always wait for another year.

Also, Ayurvedic Detox works flawlessly for all age groups. There is no age factor involved. But the younger you are, the faster the process will occur. There are also Ayurvedic *Rasayanas* which can be used during this process.

Rasayanas are Ayurvedic formulations that help post detoxification process. However, they must be consumed as directed by the physician, or as mentioned in the product. If you are planning to take any of these measures, it is better you consult a physician. They are considered to provide a healing benefit to the person.

There are many types of Ayurvedic diets and the detox diet is just one of them. Please keep in mind not to consider, or mix up any other Ayurvedic diet that you come across from other sources. We do not recommend you doing that, but in case you do, please make sure that they are Ayurvedic Detox diets or recipes.

There might be different methods of detox, but the most common one is to follow these three phases. That is what we recommend. There are also week by week, day by day and other types of cleansing cycles that could be followed. That is up to you, but it is not very necessary.

So, are you ready to get cleansed? Let's get those toxins out of your body. But before that, let's get you to know a little about Ayurveda.

Vedic Living

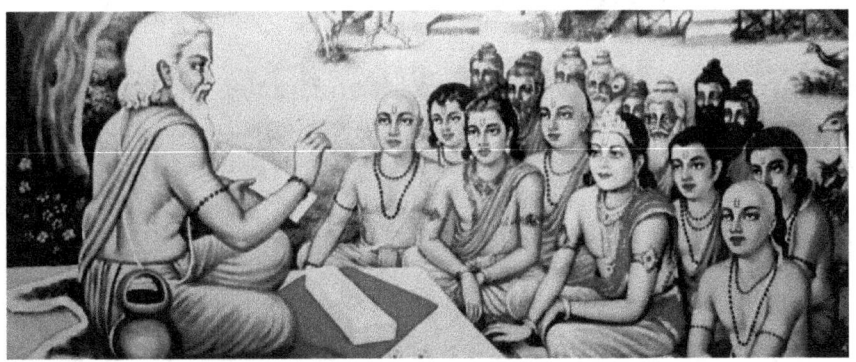

Source: vedicartandscience.com

Ayurvedic Detox processes are normally based on the Vedic lifestyle. The Vedic lifestyle evolved from the 'Vedas', who were once part of Ancient India. Vedic living can also be accredited to Hinduism and Hindu teachings, and it is where the religion evolved from.

Vedic living or the Vedic culture stresses on spirituality, and that is a very important aspect of Ayurveda. But experts believe that the Vedic culture was a 'way of living' rather than just a religion.

The Vedic culture involves a lot of rites, and customary traditions. That goes into the history books, and if you are interested to learn a lot about them, you could go ahead. But guess what, the Vedic Living style is not so important to follow the Ayurvedic Detox, except for a few general things.

The real truth is that the Vedic style of living cannot be actually defined. We do not know what the people have been doing, and the little things that the researches understood were only through the clues obtained from the things they left behind.

However, the Vedic culture does not have a specific God or a prophet, like most religions. It is completely different and very much complex when compared to the Western religions. That is one reason why we cannot talk much about it. On the other hand, you are here to detox your body, and not to concentrate on the Vedic way of living.

But there is one thing you have to learn. The Vedic living style was highly disciplined. When undergoing Ayurvedic Detox discipline is very essential. Here are a few things that explain the Vedic living style. This will also help us to understand why Ayurvedic Detox is very important. Here goes:

- Vedic Living is based on a philosophy of Universal Spiritual truths, called Sanatana-Dharma.

- Based on the belief that the 'Supreme Being' resides in the heart of all living things, the Vedic style of living gives us the idea that anyone can achieve anything.

- 'Karma' is something that evolved from the Vedic philosophy. Whatever you do, comes back to you, no matter whether it is good or bad. This normally means "Do good, receive good".

- People follow Vedic culture and strict rules to gain 'spiritual identity'.

- The Vedic literature is the basis of the Vedic living lifestyle. This is followed in most Hindu scriptures till date. These books are believed to be "Non ordinary". It is believed that they were written by some force, and not a human being.

- Cleanliness is a very important aspect of living, and it is the duty of every human to be clean and follow his cleanliness procedures.

- Peace, firmness, forgiveness, self control, avoiding dishonesty, intelligence, knowledge, truthfulness, control over the five senses, and anger management are the important aspects of a righteous life.

These are the basics of the Vedic life that you should understand. You could very well do more research on this, but it is not needed.

The Three Doshas of Ayurveda

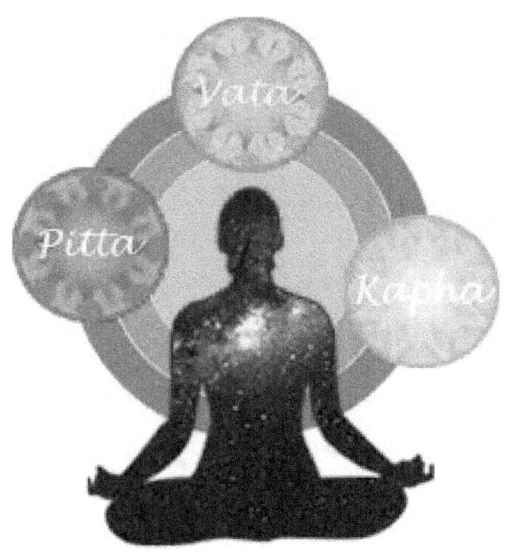

Source: www.alternalive.net

The main idea of Ayurveda is that every person on Earth is unique. That is what all scientists would agree to as well. According to Ayurveda, there is no specific diet, and every person can follow the one that suits him best. In other words, this is the specialty of this medicine.

Ayurveda also sticks on to the old proverb, which says "Prevention is better than cure". The best thing about Ayurvedic Detox is that it is completely natural. There is no medicine involved and it does not induce any artificial system to your body. There are also no side effects at all.

If you are wondering what Doshas are, do not get confused. If you have been to India, towards the South, one of the most staple foods is Dosa. But in Ayurveda, Dosha means energy. There are 3 Doshas in Ayurveda, which represent the 3 energies. They are known as Vata Dosha, Pitta Dosha and Kapha Dosha.

Vata Dosha

Ayurveda is based on self control. In many cases, people who have diseases that cannot be treated, go to Ayurvedic doctors. They are counselled to accept their condition and live with it. Vata Dosha controls bodily functions which are related to motion. "Vata"means circle. This includes blood circulation, breathing, blinking, and heartbeat.

Pitta Dosha

Ayurveda is an old method, but still, people were clever enough to understand metabolism. Pitta Dosha is the energy which controls the metabolism of a human body. Digestion, absorption, nutrition, and body temperature are controlled using Pitta Dosha.

Kapha Dosha

This is something that every living being undergoes. Kapha Dosha is the energy that controls the growth in a human being's body. It is also believed that Kapha Dosha is the energy that helps I water supply. There are many positive and negative effects of these energies.

But even if all these Doshas are present in an individual, the philosophy of Ayurveda states that only 1 or 2 Doshas will be dominantly available in an individual. The dominant Dosha is determined with the help of personal traits.

If you are thin, tall, creative, lively and full of energy, then you have the Vata energy predominant in you. You will also hate cold climate and love hot climate. You will have dry skin, and you will not sweat much. You will also have mood swings often.

If you are of a medium, well built physique, then you are a pitta predominant type. You will have a sharp concentration and strong ideas. However, you will also be very aggressive. You will have a strong appetite. Beyond all this, you will have a great leadership ability.

If you have a very strong and hefty physique, then you are a Kapha predominant type. You will also be calm, soft spoken, and you can get easily depressed. You want to be peaceful and maintain peace, while you also expect other people in your surroundings to do the same.

These are the types of Doshas that people can determine. Which Dhosa is yours?

Why Do We Have To Detox?

Our body detoxifies itself through sweat and other types of excretion, but during the winter season, we do not excrete much. Hence, all these toxins accumulate in our bodies. On the other hand, toxins can also get accumulated in our bodies because of the environment. Polluting agents will lodge in our bodies, and the massive industrialization has made us prone to these problems. There are different types of toxins that every human being will have, and detoxifying is important in order to get rid of them.

Different Types of Toxins

The major toxins of the human body can be classified into two types. They are the exogenous and endogenous toxins. As the names suggest, exogenous toxins are the ones which come from the outside and endogenous toxins are the ones that come from the inside. They are also further classified as follows.

Exogenous Toxins

Exogenous toxins come from environmental pollution as well as consumption. All types of bad habits like smoking, drinking, drugs and inhalation or exposure to harmful stuff like heavy metals are caused by exogenous toxins. Emotional factors are also included in Exogenous toxins.

Air pollution is a major element of exogenous toxins. Climate change, sudden climate shifts, global warming, exposure to radiation, all these are also part of exogenous toxins. Pesticides in food, fertilizers, herbicides, etc. are all chemically manufactured these days. This is why it is very important to follow an organic diet during the detox process.

Drinking water and food are also the simplest agents of exogenous toxins. It is very, very essential that you take care of this. Water is not at all natural these days. Whether you drink water from the tap or from packaged water bottles, they also contain preservatives and other chemicals.

Your house is one of the most unavoidable agents of exogenous toxins. It is essential that you keep your house as clean as possible. Even when it is clean, you will be exposed to toxins, but the level will be minimized.

Try not to stress yourself. The more you stress, the more toxins you will create. Though this creates endogenous toxins, stress is considered as an external agent in Ayurveda. In other words, you can control it by yourself.

Endogenous Toxins

Endogenous toxins are those toxins which occur as a result of your metabolic activities. Yes, as it was mentioned earlier, your body produces its own toxins.

Digestion is the first producer of endogenous toxins. When we eat food substances, it is converted to energy, and food is burnt. Similar to an automobile where the burnt fossil fuels produce harmful products, our body also produces exogenous toxins when it burns food.

There are also bacteria and yeast living in your intestinal tracts. These help in digestion, but at the same time, they also produce toxins. Hence, it is another source of endogenous toxins.

Since you now know the different types of toxins, it is now time to get detoxed.

Pre Cleansing Phase

The pre cleaning phase is where you get prepared for the detox process. Normally, a proper pre cleaning phase in Ayurvedic Detox requires 3 to 5 days of cleansing. If you do not drink coffee or tea, and if you do not have any habits like smoking or drinking, you can just undergo a pre cleansing phase for three days. In other words, you should be a teetotaler to undergo the pre cleansing phase for just 3 days.

But if you are not, you will have to go through 5 days of pre cleansing. However, this is recommended even for teetotalers to have a better pre cleansing effect.

The Keys to a Successful Ayurvedic Cleanse

Start with external stuff

When going through the pre cleansing phase, there are many things that you will have to come through. First, clean your surroundings and start with external stuff. Avoid going out and visiting polluted areas. Relieve yourself of stress and keep your mind clean. Meditate every day for some time.

Avoid drinking beverages except green tea. You should drink a lot of water. A minimum of 3 liters of water consumption is required every day. Also, while you consume water, drink it separately. Do not mix it with any of the other food substances. Follow all the procedures carefully.

However, when you begin with detox, do not start everything all of a sudden. Start slowly and work your way up gradually. If you stress yourself too much, it will lead to a lot of problems.

Decluttering tips:

Here are a few decluttering tips:

- Use dairy substitutes such as hemp, rice, and nut milks. Non gluten grains are also good. Avoid any food which involves gluten and other substances.

- Consume a lot of fruits and vegetables. However, make sure that all of them are organic. Genetically modified fruits and vegetables will only increase the toxins.

- Take a lot of vegetable protein and animal protein. Vegetable protein is more recommended.

- Green vegetables are good for decluttering. These are the very important foods or the pre cleansing stage.

- Avoid fatty substances. Use sunflower oil, olive oil or flax seed oil instead. Any seed oil can be used.

- Drink a lot of herbal tea or green tea. Avoid coffee and other beverages.

- Filtered water, mineral water, and seltzer should be consumed well.

- Instead of artificial sweeteners or sugar, use brown rice syrup, stevia, natural fruits and dried fruits.

Avoid These:

- Avoid dairy products, soybean, pork, beef, and any canned food.

- Never ever eat peanuts or peanut butter.

- Avoid eating chocolate, coconuts, bananas, and strawberries.

- Butter, cheese and mayonnaise should also not be consumed.

- Eggs should also be avoided. Bread items, and any of those with a high protein dose should also be avoided.

Are you ready to go through the pre cleansing stage? Let's give it a go! It is not that difficult, but it will take some time to get accustomed to it. Try your best to follow the above tips for the next 5 days. But once you decide to do it, never give up!

The Cleanse Phase

If you have successfully completed your cleanse phase, then it is time to enter the cleanse phase. This is where you will be strictly following the Kitchari mono diet. And by strict, we mean real strict. If you are wondering what on earth the Kitchari Monodiet is, do not worry, it will be explained in the next paragraph.

What is Kitchari Monodiet?

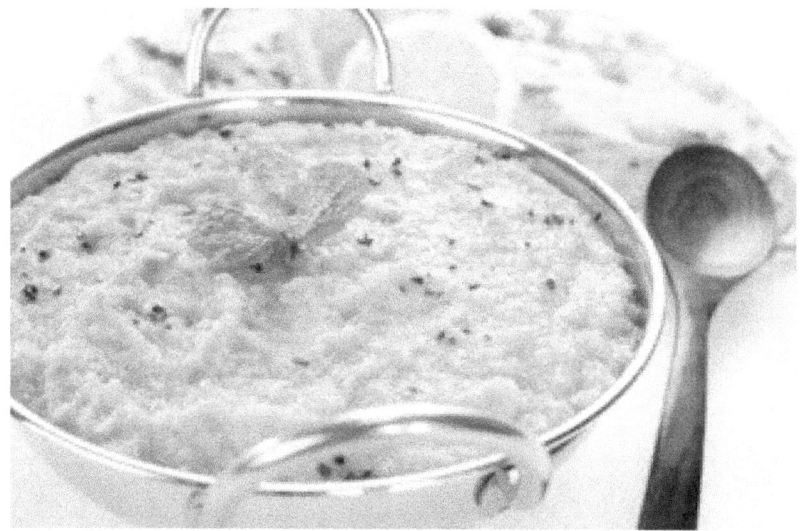

Source: beyondgoodhealthclinics.com.au

The Kitchari Monodiet is an ancient detox diet. The truth is that even scientists could not find diet so nutritious that this diet is pretty famous today. You might be thinking what a mono diet means? It is nothing complicated. It detoxifies the digestive system, and it is one of the easiest foods to make.

Kitchari actually means 'porridge'. This is an Indian term used for it. People go with the Kithcari diet because it is very useful or detox, and at the same time, it also provides nutrition. While undergoing detox, you will be under a diet, and this will lead to a lot of problems. One of them is lack of nutrition.

When you take the Kitchari mono diet, you will eat the same food two to three times a day. Nothing else should be consumed in between. The main ingredient of Kitchari is "Dal", which is known as "lentils" in English. There are many Kitchari recipes, out of which a few are mentioned here.

Simple Katchari Recipe

This is a recipe for lazy people. If you are lazy and don't mind about the taste of your Katchari, then you can stick on to this.

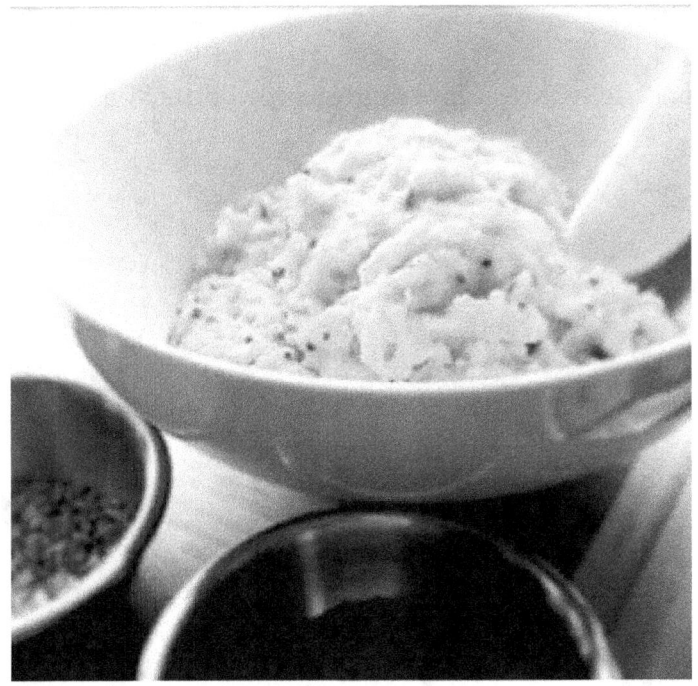

Source: instatagphoto.com

Ingredients:

1 cup basmati rice
1 cup yellow split mung dal
1 small handful cilantro leaves, chopped
6 cups water

Instructions:

Wash the dal and soak it for a few hours before cooking. Add the other ingredients to the water and stir well. Bring to a boil for 5 minutes. Turn the heat to a low,and wait for half an hour. Stir occasionally. You can eat it hot.

Plain Kitchari Recipe

This is another plain recipe, but it tastes better than the previous one.

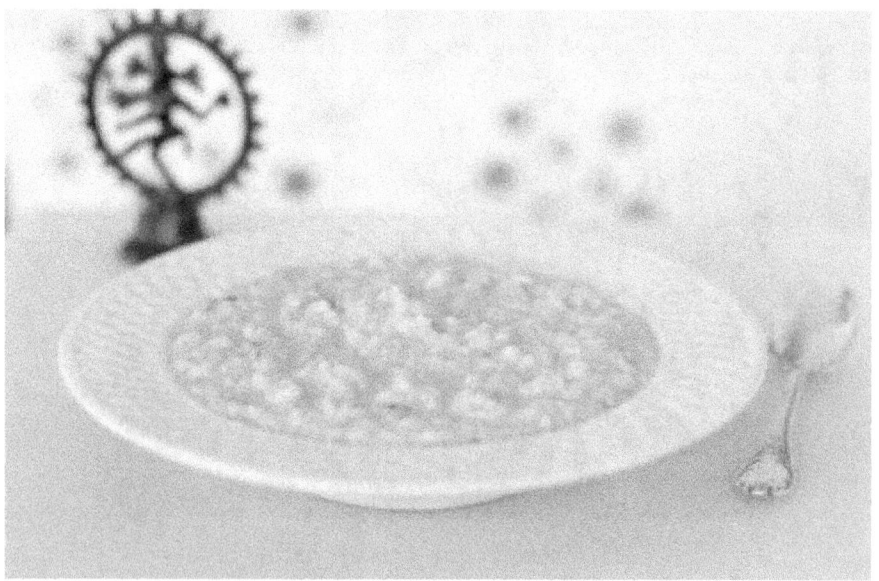

Source: shirleytwofeathers.blogspot.com

Ingredients:

1/4 cup basmati rice
1/4 cup mung beans
1 cup water
1 tablespoon yogurt or kefir
A pinch of sea salt
1 tablespoon butter or ghee, or virgin coconut oil

Instructions:

All the rice and the beans in a pot with yoghurt, and mix well. Add water and soak overnight. Bring to a boil, stir well and then reduce the flame to a low. Add salt, ghee or any other alternative 5 minutes before removing from the heat and stir well.

Spicy Kitchari Recipe

This is the spiciest Kitchari recipe you can ever make.

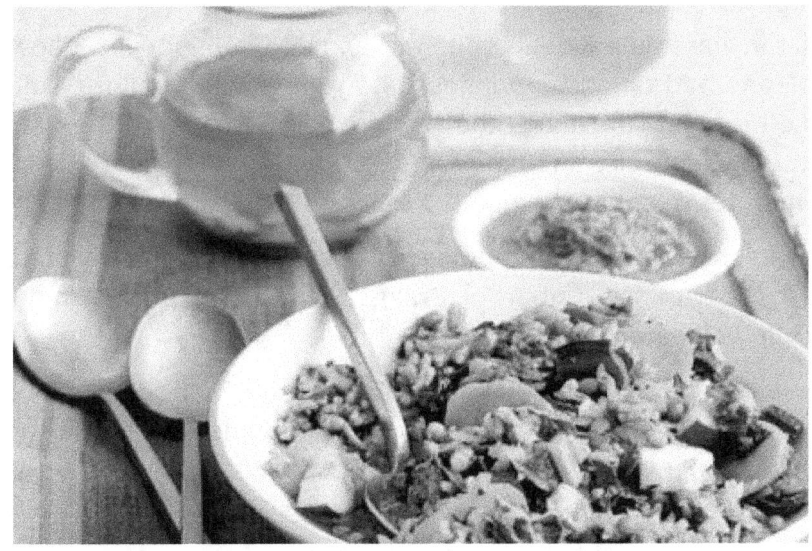

Source: www.yogajournal.com

Ingredients:

4 quarts water
1 cup mung beans, sorted and rinsed well
2 medium onions, chopped
2" piece ginger root, peeled and finely chopped
2 teaspoons turmeric
1/2 teaspoon ground black pepper
1/2 teaspoon ground cardamom
3/4 teaspoon cumin seeds
2 teaspoons curry powder or garam masala
2 tablespoons minced garlic
6 cups chopped assorted vegetables
1 1/4 cups basmati rice, sorted and rinsed well
2 tablespoons butter or ghee
Salt, tamari soy sauce or Bragg Liquid Aminos to taste

Instructions:

Boil the water in a 6 quart soup pot and add mung beans. Allow to cook and add onions and ginger later on. Now add all the spices. At one point of time, the beans will split, and the garlic, vegetables and rice should be added then. Allow to cook for 15 to 20 minutes over high flame.

Stir well occasionally. Add butter or ghee, and then slowly start to season it with salt, tamari or Braggs. Allow to set for 15 minutes and sir well before eating.

These are the best recipes for your Kitchari Monodiet, and you can also try all three of them. But this diet, which is also known as the Kitchari Cleanse, is not a useless one. It will start working immediately.

The Kitchari Monodiet should be followed strictly. DO not eat anything else. Normally, it is advised at the Kitchari Monodiet should be consumed 2-3 times a day. This will make it more effective.

If you have a good Yoga center nearby, you can try out some asanas early in the morning. This will help in a better state of mind, and yoga has also been accredited with accelerating he detox process. However, there are a few problems too.

When you follow the Kitchari Monodiet, you might sometimes fall victim to constipation. This might happen if you had reduced your water intake. Water is very essential for detox. It increases the amount of fluids in the body, and this is very essential, because during detox, most of the metabolic systems and other systems are altered.

This is induced naturally, but still, it is induced. Hence the body needs more water. Beets and sprouts can be added to the Kitchari Monodiet if you are constipated. The best remedy is radish sprouts. Some people recommend banana as bananas, but it is not at all advised when going through detox.

4 Day Pre Cleanse With Internal Oleation

During the first 4 days of the Cleanse program, the Kitchari Monodiet will be followed 2 to 3 times a day. But this is accompanied with another procedure called Internal Oleation. This is known as *Snehana* in Ayurveda. Oleation can be internal or external, but internal oleation has the most benefits. This is called as *Snehapanam*, which means intake of oils.

You might have noted that ghee or some other oil would have been added in every recipe of Kitchari Monodiet. The reason for adding these is because of internal oleation. But apart from adding these in food substances, ghee and oil can also be consumed directly.

2-3 tablespoons of ghee can be consumed two times every day during the cleansing stage. This will increase fluids in your body and avoid problems like constipation. You can also drink a lot of green tea or Ayurvedic herbal tea.

1 Day Rest

After the 4 day cleanse period is over, you will feel a bit tired. This is when you will have to rest well. Eat a lot of organic fruits and drink juice cleanses. These are mostly green smoothies. They will rejuvenate our energy, and at the same time help you to get some new taste. The taste buds will be bored of the same Kitchari Monodiet.

Different Types of Traditional Ayurvedic Cleanse Diet

Here are a few other diets that help in the cleanse stage, in case you hate the Kitchari Monodiet very badly.

Rice Water (Manda)

The only two things you will need for this recipe are rice and water.

Ingredients:

Rice
Water

Instructions:

The ratio is very important here. You will have to add 2 tablespoons of rice to one cup of water. Boil well until the rice becomes very tender. Remove the rice, and now you have rice water. If it is too thick, then add some more water and make it thin. It can be refrigerated, heated and reused. So do not worry about the quantity at all.

Rice Soup (Peya)

Peya is another important recipe that will help during the Cleansing stage. This is otherwise known as the rice soup or Chinese rice soup.

Ingredients:

1 cup basmati rice
16 cups water
1 teaspoon ghee
1 tablespoon marjoram
1 tablespoon lovage
1 tablespoon chervil
1 tablespoon parsley
4 pinches ground coriander
4 pinches ground cumin
1 pinch asafetida
Salt

Instructions:

Mix the rice and the water and cook on medium heat in a pot for 15 minutes. Stir and whisk while cooking. On the other hand, heat the ghee with spices in a skillet. Ladle some of the soup into the skillet and allow to cook well.

After some time, put it back in the rice pot. Reduce he heat and wait for the rice to become tender. When the soup is ready, add the herbs and salt to taste.

Thick Rice Soup (Vilepi)

Vilepi, which is also known as thick rice soup is served with 4 parts of water to 1 part of basmati rice. The preparation same as the other soups, but basmati rice is used. Sugarcane powder, ginger, garlic, turmeric, and ghee can also be added.

Cooked Rice (Odana)

Read that as Odana, not Obama. Cooked rice can be made from soups. It is simple. You will just have to eat the filtered rice instead of throwing it out. The rice normally cannot be eaten alone, but you can eat it with salt. That makes it a bit edible. Also, you can add a little water and curd/yoghurt to it. This will help in better consumption of the Cooked Rice. It is a very good food for stamina.

Mung Dal Soup (Yusha)

Add some Mung Dal to Peya (rice soup+), and then you will get the Yusha. Mung Dal is again added as an ingredient for extra strength. Mung Dal Soup is said to make the taste better as well. It is also added in most Ayurveda recipes.

Kitchari

The Kitchari diet has been previously explained and you can find 3 types of Kitchari recipes in the table of contents section.

Food Guidelines According to the Three Doshas

Do you remember the 3 Doshas? They might look simple,but the 3 doshas have a great significance in Ayurveda. If you haven't found your dosha yet, it is high time you did, because you will only get the perfect detox benefits when you find the right Dosha.

Food Guidelines for Vata Dosha

- Consume more quantities of food. But make it a point that you do not eat too much.

- Consume at least 3 teaspoons of ghee daily throughout the detox process. This can be done either directly or indirectly.

- Natural sweeteners can also be consumed for people who have vata dosha.

- Light dairy products can be consumed. Warm milk is one of the best products and they are easier to be consumed when warm.

- Rice and wheat are the most important grains to be consumed. Barley, corn, millet, buckwheat, and rye should be avoided.

- Avoid eating light fruits. Apple, pears and pomegranates should be avoided. Heavy fruits and dry fruits can also be eaten.

- You must not eat raw vegetables. Only cooked vegetables are the best for you.

- Gas producing food products must be avoided.

- Spices and nuts are very good for vata dosha.

- Beans must be avoided, however, you can at mung beans.

Food Guidelines for Pitta Dosha

- Dairy products like milk, butter and ghee can be used. Yogurt, sour cream and cheese typically, any dairy product which is sour, should be avoided.

- Molasses and Honey are not good for you. Other sweeteners are allowed. Green vegetables and leafy vegetables are recommended.

- Wheat, rice, barley, and oats are the best grains. Reduce the consumption of corn, rye, millet, and brown rice.

- Try to use cool and soothing seasonings. Hot seasonings should be reduced or completely avoided.

- Eat fennel seeds after consumption of normal meals. This will reduce the acidic reactions in the stomach.

Food Guidelines for Kapha Dosha

- Fresh vegetables and fruit juices are the best foods. A liquid fat once a week during the cleanse stage is recommended.

- Avoid all dairy products except ghee. The others are not advised.

- You can only use honey as a sweetener. You can drink 1 tablespoon of raw honey every day. However, do not cook with honey, since it would be a disaster.

- Avoid soybean. All other beans are good to go.

- Lighter fruits must be consumed. Avoid heavy fruits. These would definitely be a disaster.

- Vegetables are very good for Kapha Dosha. However, you must avoid eating tomatoes, zucchini, and sweet potatoes.

- Dinner must be as light as possible. A 3 hour gap is essential before going to bed.

- You should drink hot ginger tea after meals. This will help in digestion.

Thus, if you follow these food guidelines according to your doshas, you will get a better chance of detoxification.

If you're liking this book so far I would really appreciate it if you could stop at the Kindle store and leave a review and a rating for it.

Please take a second to go to the Amazon page and leave a review if you found some good pointers about the gluten free lifestyle.

Thank you so very, very much for buying my book.

Post Cleanse Detox Practices

Once you have undergone the detox process, you will have to start getting back to your normal life. Post cleansed detox practices are very essential, since you will have to main a proper diet and make the best out of your detox process. Neglecting it will result in a huge problem.

These are a few tips that one will have to follow post detox.

To Eat:

- Eat easily digestible foods. During detox, the digestive system I completely modified and it will take time for it to get back to normal. You might feel like there is a stone in your stomach. This is because of eating food that was not easily digested.

- Do not overeat. After detox, most people do not feel very hungry, but they still stuff themselves with food. Never ever do that. You should eat only when you are hungry.

- Vegetables that could be easily digested should be on your list for some time during the post detox stage. There are many other Ayurvedic recipes that are included towards the end of the book, but it is suggested that you avoid non vegetarian foods.

- Vegetables are easier to digest, and hence more experts recommend this. You should take vegetables for at least a week after detox.

- Mild spices can be added in your diet. According to Ayurveda, spices are good for detox. They also improve the taste of your food. In case you strained them too much, the taste buds might be longing for something that tastes good, and that is where mild spices will help.

Not to Eat:

- Avoid common allergens like wheat, soy, corn, dairy, peanuts and walnuts.

- Tomatoes, white potatoes, eggplants, peppers and sweet potatoes should be avoided.

- Avoid broccoli, cauliflower, cabbage and Brussels sprouts. Any type of sprouts will cause gas in the stomach, and they all need to be seriously avoided.

- Avoid heavy dairy products.

- Heavy spices should also be avoided.

- Always say no to processed food.

- Avoid drinking coffee or anything that contains caffeine. If you cannot survive without coffee, then try drinking decaffeinated coffee.

If you start practicing this for a few days, you will lose the cravings for processed foods. Take a vacation or visit some place which is serene, to relax your body and your mind. Do not give you your diet under any circumstances.

If you keep following this, you will slowly get to make this as your default diet. You will stop all your bad habits, and will slowly reduce the amount of toxins that you take in. The basic principle of Ayurveda is that the body will heal itself.

If you keep following this diet after detox or the post cleanse phase, you will get stronger, and your healing power will further improve. Detox is not something that happens once. You will have to undergo regular cleansing in order to stay fit.

You can eat the foods you like once a while. There is no harm in doing it, but do it very, very rarely.

Detox Tips for the Post Cleanse Period

During the post cleanse period, you can be easy on your diet, but there are few recipes that will help you get through this phase easily.

Hot Lemon Water

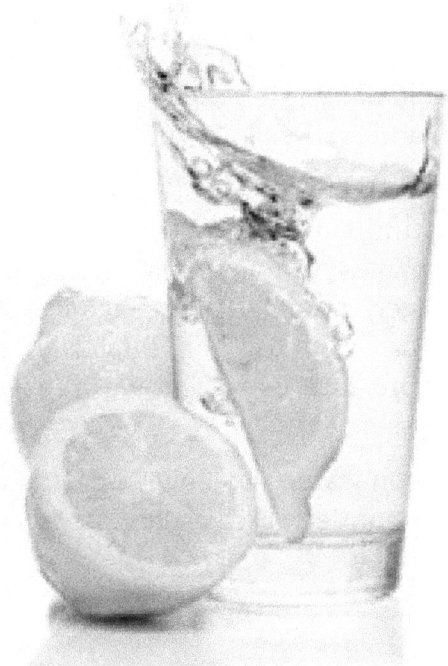

Source: www.mypurebalance.ca

Making lemon water is not a big deal. You will just have to squeeze a few drops of lemon in hot or warm water. But the time of drinking this is very important. Most Ayurveda experts recommend that you must drink lemon water early in the morning, on an empty stomach.

Though this is not the only time, you can also drink it before going to bed, but it has a good effect when consumed in the mornings.

Benefits:

Lemon water helps in digestion. Hot water itself normally helps in digestion, but adding lemon to it increases the benefits. Lemon water can also be consumed to rejuvenate your energy. It also helps with hydration.

Whether you follow an Ayurvedic diet or not, lemon water is an essential element in all walks of life. It also acts as a natural flush. In other words, it cleans your stomach and the digestive system. If you start drinking lemon water regularly, you will have better bowel movement, and you will also be void of constipation and other problems.

Lemon also boosts the immune system. Apart from that, it also has cosmetic advantages. Lemon water is rich in vitamin C, and this helps in collagen production. Collagen helps in smooth, healthy skin. You can also use the squeezed lemon zests by applying them to your face when you wash it. This will help in providing a glowing skin.

Apart from this, lemon water also helps a person concentrate on his weight. It reduces or decreases weight according to your body type.

Scams:

There are many websites on the internet claiming that lemon water will cure cancer, balance pH level and increase IQ. All these claims are very much fake.

Daily Bowel Movement

Bowel movement is very important in order to facilitate digestion. Proper bowel movements always help in maintaining a clean digestive system. Your stool should neither be too hard or too loose. If it is too hard, then you are experiencing constipation, and if it is too loose, then you are experiencing diarrhea or loose motion.

There are a few techniques to be followed to have proper bowel movements. They are as follows.

- Eat more fiber oriented foods. Beans, fresh fruits and vegetables are rich in fiber. Constipation is only due to lack of fiber.

- Lemon water is very good for bowel movements. Not just lemon water, but water itself is a very good agent for proper bowel movement.

- Fruit juices also help in bowel movement. Drink a lot of fruit juices. They will not only hydrate the body, but will also help in better bowel movements, thereby helping the person.

- Herbal tea or green tea also helps in bowel movements.

- Try to be stress free, stress hampers bowel movements too.

- Whenever you feel like pooping or peeing, you will have to do it, and not resist yourself.

Bowel movements can also differ based on the type of doshas, and that is why you will have to choose your dosha and follow the diet according to those guidelines.

Self Massage and its Implications

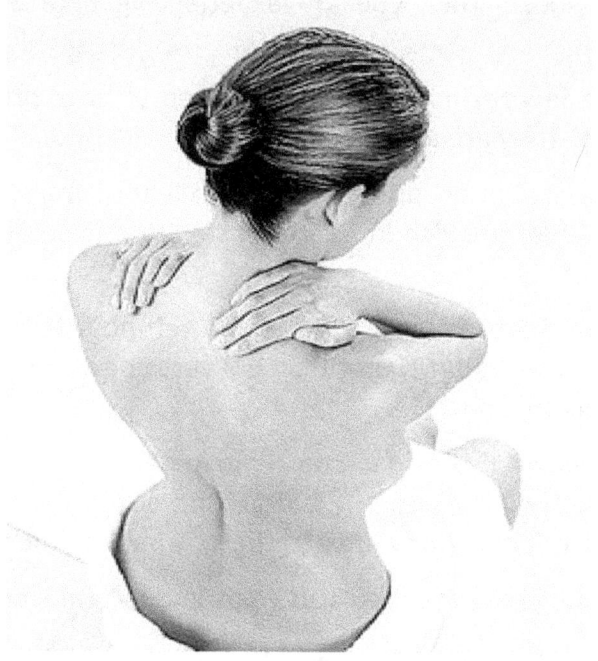

Source: vashsovet.com.ua

India is famous for its Ayurvedic massages and this is done with oil. Ayurvedic oil massage can be done by professionals, but what is more special is that it can also be done by yourself. Ayurvedic self massage is known as Abhyanga. It is a must for Vata dosha.

Abhanyga is a simple technique. You will have to apply the Ayurvedic oil to your body and allow it to soak well for quite some time. After that, you should take a hot shower. There are seven tissues in the body and according to this massage technique, all the 7 layers must be massaged.

The massage can last from a minimum of 15 minutes for a couple of hours. Applying oil to the body before massaging is also known as external oleation. There are different videos on YouTube about Ayurrvedic self massage, so you can check them out. It is much better than reading something and wondering how to practically do it.

Benefits of Self Massage:

Self massage is very essential for a person's relaxation. In one way, massage promotes relaxation, and relaxation reduces stress, thereby helping in better detox. It stimulates the internal organs of the body and also pacifies the vata and pitta doshas.

Body Massage Benefits:

Applying oil to the body increases the softness of the skin, improves the color of the skin and also makes you feel young. By color, don't think that you will become fair. Your complexion will get rich, and that's it. Body massage also improves sleep patterns and improves firmness the tissues. It also stimulates the internal organs of the body. Blood circulation and purification will also be aggravated.

Scalp Massage Benefits:

Scalp massage is known as *Murdha Taila*. Bhringaraj Oil and Brahmi Oil are used for massaging your scalp. This improves hair growth and also improves the thickness of hair. It also prevents dry scalp, dandruff and other scalp infections. Scalp massage also reduces wrinkles on your face and invigorates the sense organs.

Ear Massage Benefits:

Massaging your ear will lead to amazing benefits. It is known as *Karna Puran*. Disorders in the ear will be cleared. Ear massage also reduces stiffness in the neck and the jaw. Ear massage is also said to relieve stress and increase relaxation.

Feet Massage Benefits:

The feet are where the acupressure of the body is concentrated. The feet massage reduces the coarseness of the feet and makes it soft, it also helps to remove any cramps or dislocations. The feet will become firm and the overall circulation of the body will be increased. Feet massage is known as *padaghata*.

Dry Skin Brushing

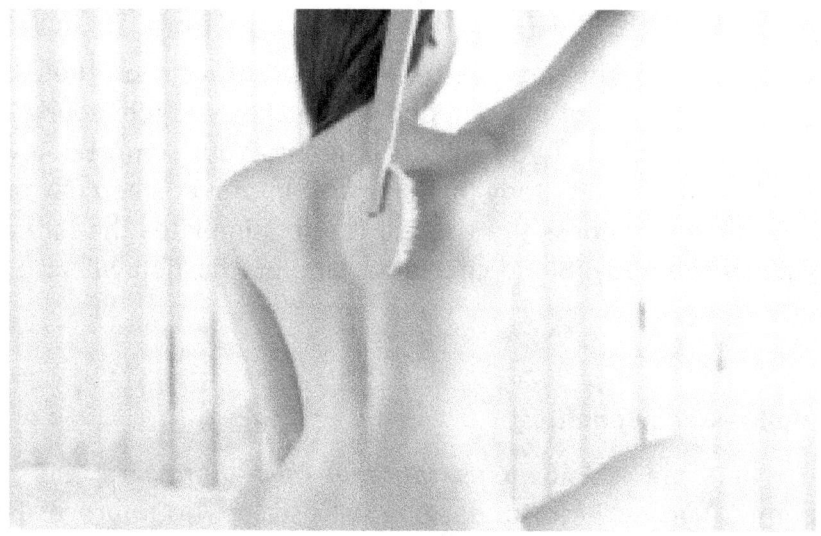

Source: beautynskincare.com

Dry Skin Brushing is another important procedure to follow post detox. Here are a few tips to do the perfect dry skin brushing.

- Buy a natural bristled brush. Also check for a long handle. This will help in greater accessibility.

- When you brush off your dry skin, it will come out of your body and fall down. It is advised that you get into a bathtub (without water) to do this.

42

- Get naked and brush the dry skin thoroughly. Do not even spare one part of your body.

- Start with your feet. Bush well, and apply little pressure, brushing the area for some time.

- Take your own time. The more you brush, the better the results.

- While you are brushing, begin with the feet and slowly progress upwards.

- Sensitive areas must be taken care of. However, you will slowly get used to the process.

- After you are done brushing, take a warm shower. A shower with varied temperature will enhance circulation.

- After you are done showering, dry yourself with a towel and apply some fruit oil.

- Clean the brush with soap and dry it in the sun to kill the germs.

- Check the results after one month.

Benefits:

- Dead skin will be naturally exfoliated. Your skin will become smoother and brighter.

- The lymphatic system will be stimulated. While this will remove toxins from your body, it will also stimulate circulation.

- Cellulite will also be reduced by dry brushing. It is a natural method of removing fat trapped under the skin. In other words, it is natural liposuction.

- The pores of your skin are cleansed and the dirt from the pores are removed. This increases with time, and if you start doing this daily, your pores will always be lean. There is no need of any deep cleansing face wash or lotion.

Deep Breathing Exercises

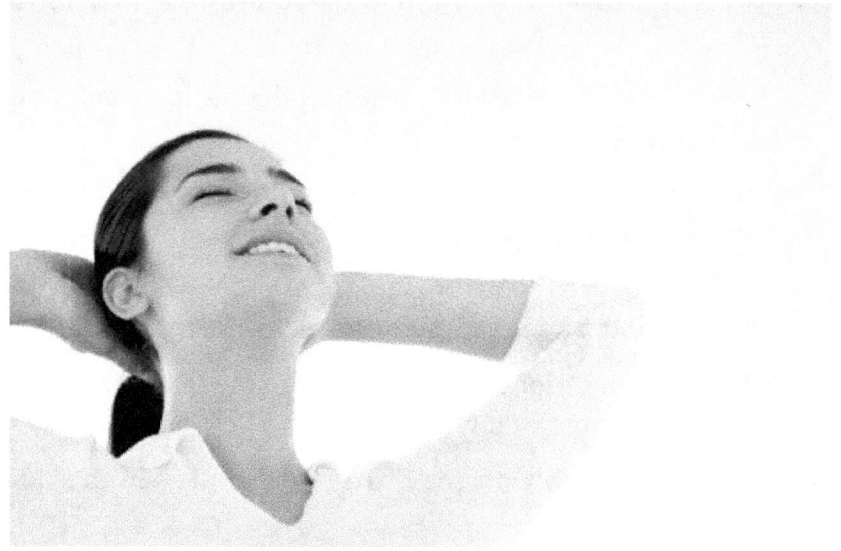

Image: healthland.time.com

Deep breathing exercises are the best remedies in Ayurveda for relaxation. Controlled breathing helps you to relax, and at the same it also helps you in the reduction of blood pressure, increase in blood circulation and gives you a calm, positive energy.

Here are the 6 breathing exercises that are a must do during the post cleanse stage. It is much better if you do them daily.

Sama Vritti

Sama Vritti or equal breathing is a good exercise to start with. You will have to breathe in and breathe out through equal counts. Inhale for 4 counts and exhale for 4 counts. Do this for 10 to 15 minutes. If you feel this is too easy, you can increase the counts, but always remember, they must be equal. Breathe using only your nose.

Abdominal Breathing

Keep your right hand on the belly and left hand on the chest. As you breathe, your diaphragm must inflate well, thereby stretching the lungs to a maximum. Take 6- 1 breaths minute. They must be deep and slow. This must be done for 6 to 8 weeks to see the complete results. It will relieve you of stress and make you feel lighter and more active.

Nadi Shodhana or Alternate Nostril Breathing

As the name says, this breathing exercise involves alternate nostril breathing. You will have to sit in your meditative position and put your right thumb the right nostril. The left nostril will now be free and you can inhale well through it. Take a deep breath and repeat with the alternate nostril.

Nadi Shodana increases the activeness of a person. It is not just a normal relaxation breath exercise. It also increases thinking capacity and focus. It might seem easy, but this breathing exercise is quite difficult.

Kapalabhati or Skull Shining Breath

This breathing exercise is another one that would make you active. It is very difficult, but you will get accustomed to it slowly. We have no idea why they call it skull shining breath, but here I how you do it.

You will have to take a long, deep breath. Then you must take a quick breath and exhale the air with your stomach. Do this alternatively, and you are a pro!

This exercise is considered equal to drinking coffee. It will make you so active.

Progressive Relaxation

It is a common thing to stretch ourselves, or exert an relax our muscles every time we feel tired. Progressive relaxation is one such thing, but here, you also control your breath when you stretch and relax.

Stretch your muscles from starting from the lowermost part of your body, which is the legs. When you do that, you will have to inhale slowly and take long, deep breaths. Do the same for all the body parts, even your eyes.

Guided Visualization

Sit in a place which is serene. It could either be your room, or your house. Position yourself as to meditate or sit in a comfortable position. Listen to some soothing music, or anything you like and concentrate on positive things. This will increase the positive energy in your mind and it will help you go through anything that is stressful.

Once you are done, you will be full of positive energy and you can complete all your tasks very easily and quickly.

These are the best breathing exercises for a starter. However, you can buy special books on air breathing techniques and improvise on them if you feel that they are effective.

Meditation

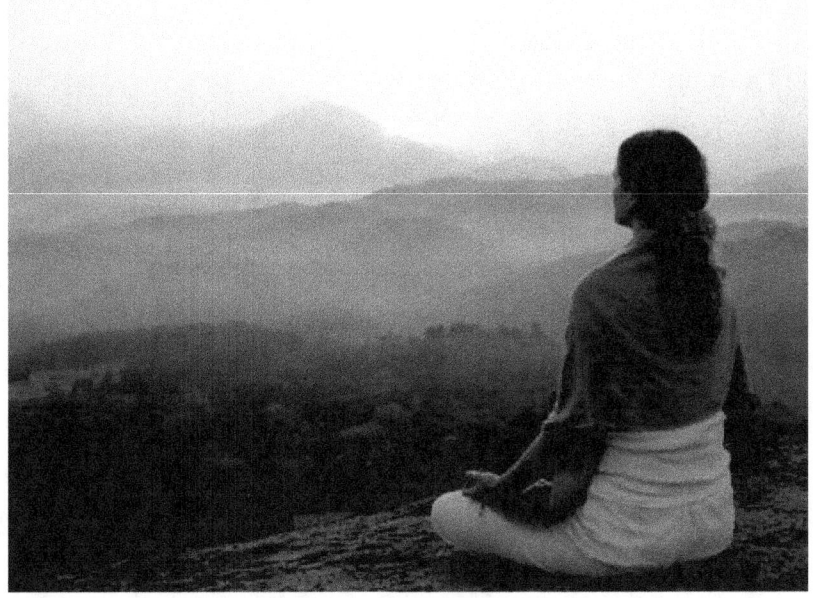

Source: anandamarga.org

Meditation is the most important form of relaxation. When you meditate, a lot of good things happen to your mind and your body. Many people have a wrong notion about meditation. When a person meditates,he is in deep thought. Meditation is more about focusing on an issue and concentrating on it.

If you just sit in some place, close your eyes and do something you like, that is not what meditation is all about. Meditation involves healing of the body and the mind. Though meditation is a very old practice, it still found it to be very effective in the 21st century.

Meditation is the only way to experience inner silence and it also helps in deep relaxation. People looking for peace of mind have to meditate well enough. Breath control during meditation also increases the benefits.

The misconception about meditation that is allows you to keep your mind quiet. The real truth, however, is the fact that meditation is the process of absorbing the quiet and the positive energy around you.

Meditation Tips

- Meditate only at a specific time and place. Normally, it is suggested that you will have to meditate early in the morning in a silent place. If your house is not silent enough, find a yoga center or a meditation center to meditate.

- It is advised that you sit up straight, close your eyes, and maintain a proper posture when you meditate.

- Breathing exercises can be followed to enhance meditation.

- Allow your mind to wander at first.

- After some time, grab some focus. This is done in order to focus naturally on something rather than focusing on it artificially.

- It will take some time to get involved in meditation. Only when you reach a state f pure thought, you will begin to forget yourself.

- Do not focus on one object, but instead focus on a category.

- This can be anything you like, and there is no restriction.

- When you lose concentration on an object, move to the other.

Sinus Cleansing

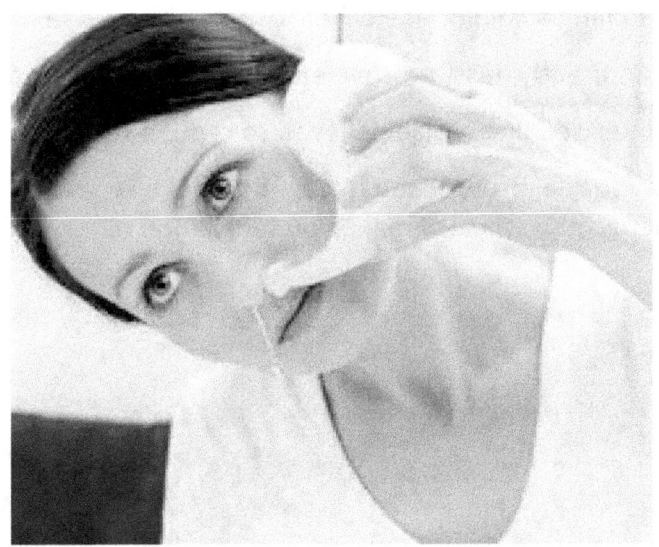

Source: www.fda.gov

This is also another essential post cleansing process. However, Sinus cleansing is not a very difficult procedure. It can be done by yourself in the very comfort of your home. You just need a few common ingredients and Neti Pot.

Mix warm water and salt and add it to the Neti Pot. GO o a wash basin or a sink. Tilt your head and insert the pot's outlet into the nasal opening which is higher. Then tilt the pot well till all the water pours in and goes out through the other nostril.

Once this is done, wipe off your nostrils with a tissue. Any type of nasal infection or any type of toxins in your nose will be cleared using the method of nasal cleansing.

Benefits:

- Sinus cleaning removes the mucus from your nose.

- Any allergins, toxins or any type of pollutant can be removed using this method in the best way.

49

- It also cleans the nose and thereby prevents you from catching a cold or any other respiratory disease.

- It indirectly has a positive effect on your breathing.

- Sinus cleaning is also believed to reduce stress.

- If you feel drowsy and heavy, this will also make you more active and will also make you feel lighter.

Oral Health

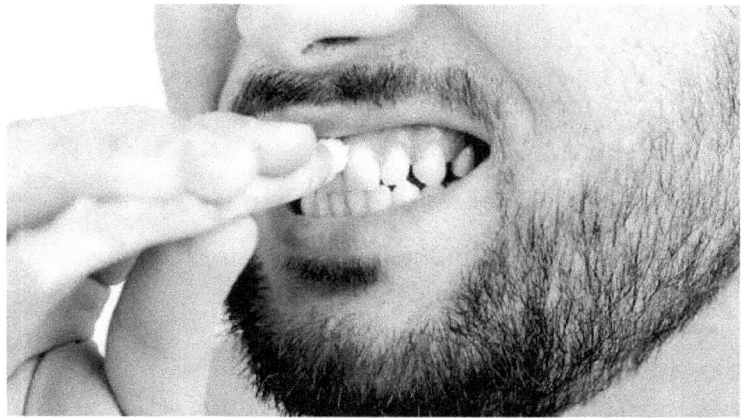

Image: www.mnn.com

Oral health is also another important phase post Ayurveda. *Danta Swasthya* is what they refer to a"Dental Health" in Ayurveda, and here are a few tips to improve it.

Chewing Sticks

Chewing sticks are not something like chewing gums. If you thought so, then you were pretty wrong. Natural sticks from plants and sticks should be chewed. There is Ayurvedic tooth paste available these days, but we recommend you to stick to the old method.

The neem stick is the most famous chewing stick. But you will also have to brush your teeth. Herbal brushes with natural bristles are available these days. This is very essential for Ayurvedic oral cleaning.

Oil Pulling

Oil Pulling is nothing but the gargling or swishing of the oil in your mouth. The most used oils for this are sesame oil ad sunflower oil. However, the most preferred one is sesame oil. Cleanse your mouth twice a day using oil to aid oil pulling. It not only cleanses the mouth, but also prevents ulcers and her infections.

Tissue Regeneration

Gum tissue regeneration is another aspect of oral care. Bilberry fruit and Hawthorne berry are the two fruits that will help in gum tissue regeneration. Other products which help in tissue regeneration include the alfalfa leaf, turmeric roots, and cinnamon barks.

Ayurvedic Breakfast Recipes

Roasted Coconut Sesame Oatmeal

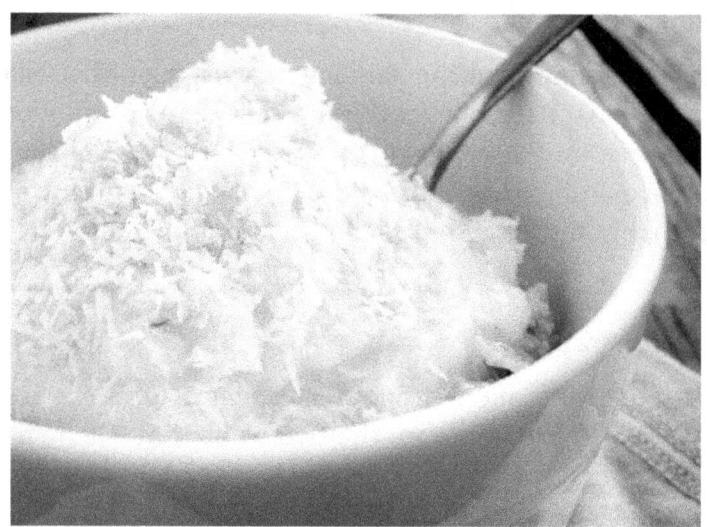

Source: www.pinterest.com

Ingredients:

3 tbsp coconut flakes
1 tbsp coconut oil
1 cup oats
1 tsp raw sugar
3 tbsp sesame seeds
3 cups water
A pinch of salt

Instructions:

Boil the water, bring the flame to a low, and then add oil and sugar. Blend or grind the oatmeal in a blender. Roast the sesame seeds and coconut shavings on medium heat. Wait until they get brown. Mix the oatmeal with cold water, add salt, and also add the oatmeal.

Stir slowly and nicely until a nice, creamy consistency is reached. Add the coconut flakes and the sesame seeds on the top before serving or eating.

Cream of Rice Soup with Ginger & Ghee

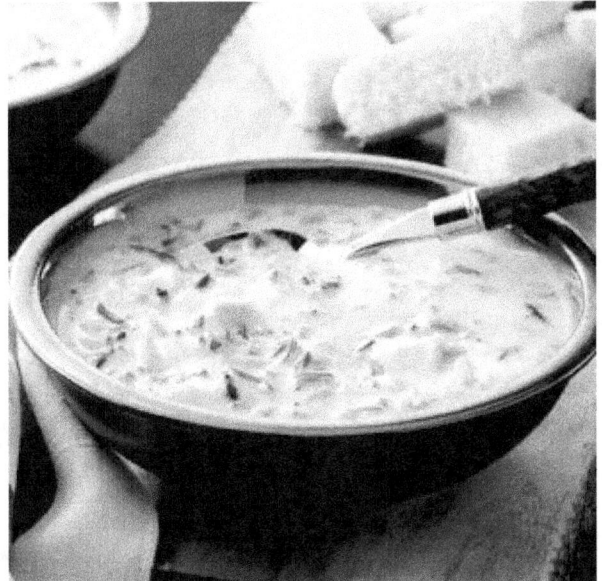

Source: www.tasteofhome.com

Ingredients:

½ cup basmati rice
¼ tsp black pepper
1 garlic clove
1 tbsp ghee

¼ inch ginger
3 cups water
Salt to taste

Instructions:

Grind the rice grains with a blender and set aside. Saute the ginger and the garlic with ghee after chopping.

Add the water and boil it. Add the rest of the ingredients and stir well, bringing them to a boil. Stir well, and serve hot.

Greens & Fresh Herb Frittata

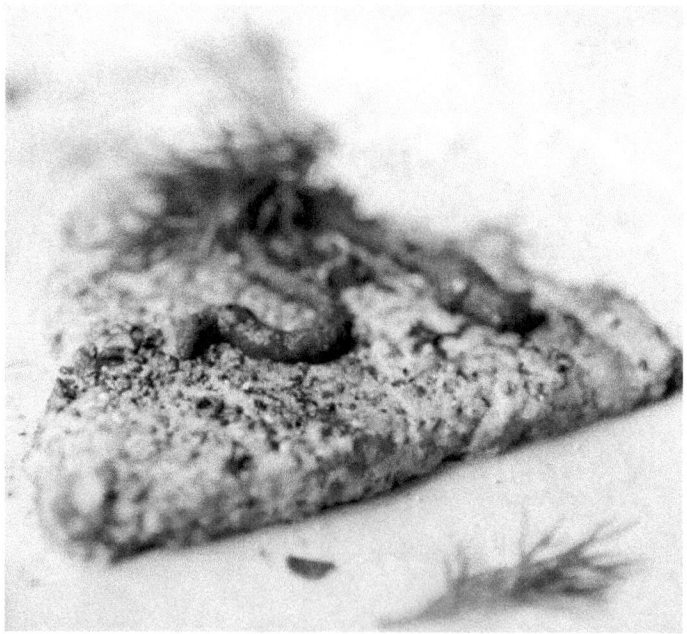

Source: kblog.lunchboxbunch.com

Ingredients:

¼ tsp black pepper

6 eggs
½ tsp oregano
1 tsp parsley
¼ tsp salt
¼ lbs spinach
1 tsp fresh thyme

Instructions:

Preheat the oven to 350 F. Cook the spinach on high heat. Whip the eggs in a bowl nicely. Chop the herbs and the spices and mix with the whipped egg.

Pour the egg in a dry sheet pan and place it in the oven.

Remove after 10 to 15 minutes.

Plum Lavender Chutney

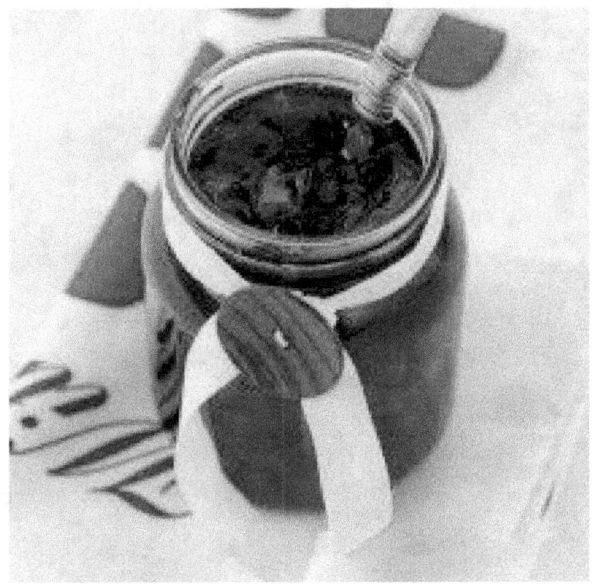

Image: www.pinterest.com

Ingredients:

½ tsp lavender
2 cups of plum
¼ tsp raw sugar

Instructions:

Skin and pit the plums. Dice the plums and set aside.

Now, mix the plums with sugar, lavender, and boil until thick.

Chill and consume whenever needed.

Morning Broth with Ghee, Lime, Salt & Spices

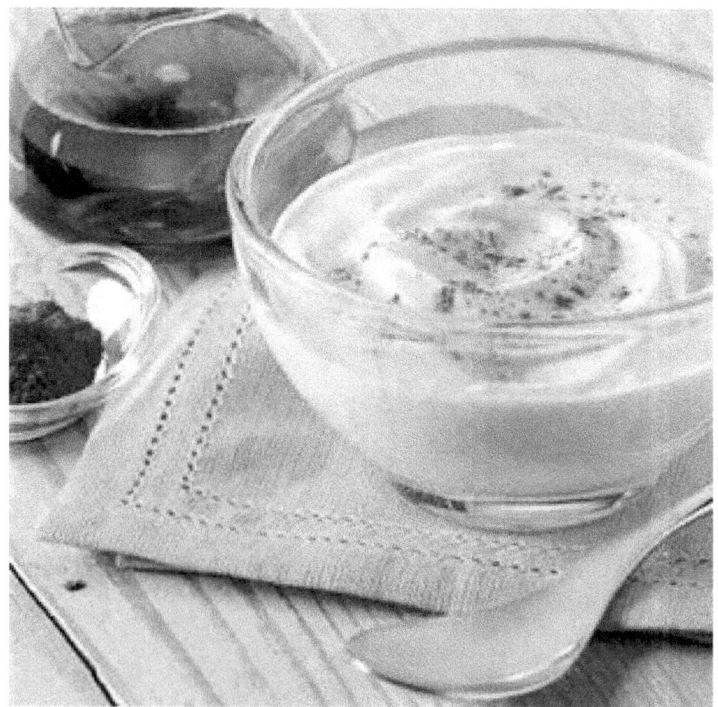

Source: www.pinterest.com

Ingredients:

2 pinches black pepper and dried ginger each
2 tbsp ghee
¼ lime
½ tsp raw sugar
2 pinches of salt

Instructions:

Boil some water. Add all the ingredients and mix well. More cups can also be made by increasing the amount and the ratio accordingly.

Ayurvedic Lunch Recipes

Quinoa with Mint, Cilantro & Red Onion

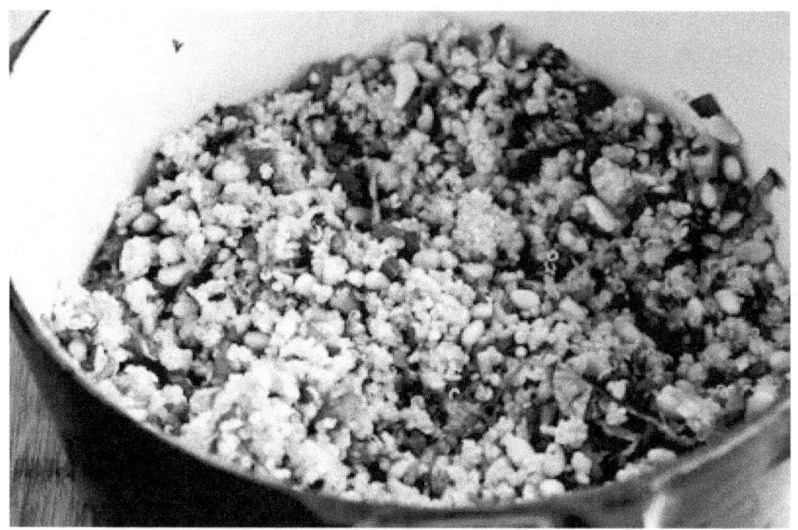

Source: www.kalynskitchen.com

Ingredients:

¼ tsp black pepper
1 cup cilantro
2 whole lime
2 tbsp mint
¼ tbsp olive oil
1 cup Quinoa
¼ cup red onion
1 tsp salt

Instructions:

Add 2 cups of water in a saucepan and boil well. Quinoa should also be added. Do not overcook, or stir too much. Chop the mint and the onions finely.

Mix all the ingredients together and serve hot.

Simple Cumin Rice

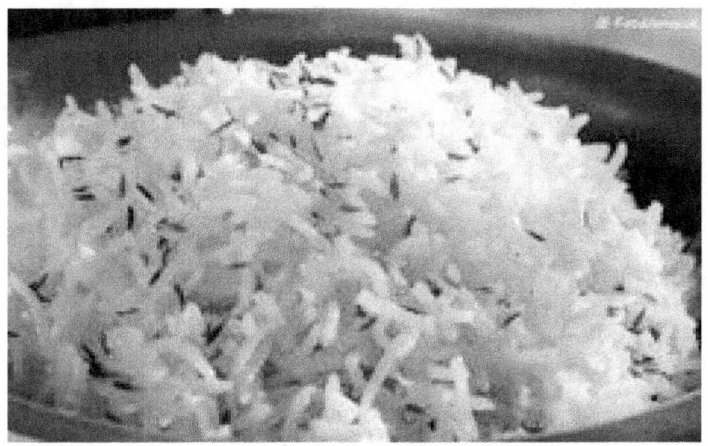

Source: www.pinterest.com

Ingredients:

1 cup of Basmati Rice
½ tsp coriander seed
½ tsp cumin
1 tsp ghee
¼ tsp salt
2 cups of water

Instructions:

Roast the cumin seeds. The roast must be dry without any addition of oil or other substances. Grind the coriander and set aside.

Now mix the salt, ground coriander, ghee, water, etc. and bring to a boil. Cover and simmer for 25 minutes.

Potatoes with Lemon and Thyme

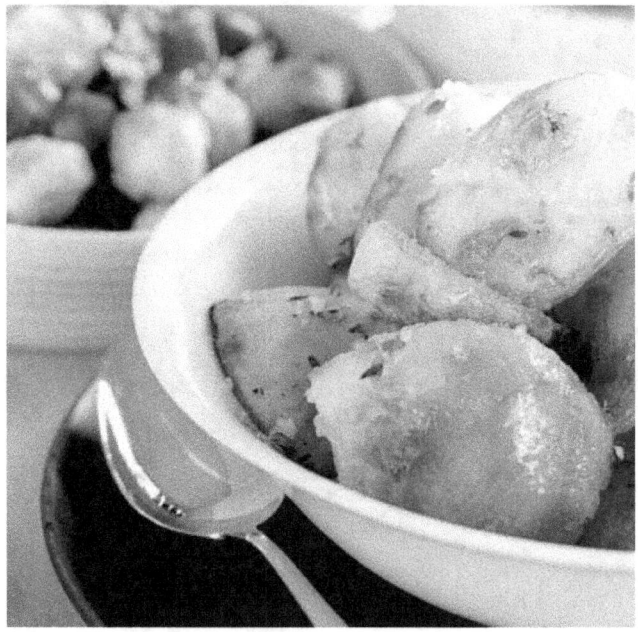

Image: www.joyfulbelly.com

Ingredients:

1 Bay Leaf
2 pinches of Black pepper
½ lemon
2 potatoes

2 pinches of salt
1 tbsp of sunflower oil
1 tbsp thyme

Instructions:

Peel the potatoes after soaking them in hot water. Mix the potato, salt, bay leaf, and black pepper in a pot with 1 cup of water. Steam well until the potatoes are cooked.

Dice the potatoes into bite sized pieces and saute well in sunflower oil. Chop the thyme and sprinkle over it. Once the potatoes become brown, remove them from the heat.

Finally, squeeze the lemon juice and mix well before eating.

Rice with Carrots & Zucchini

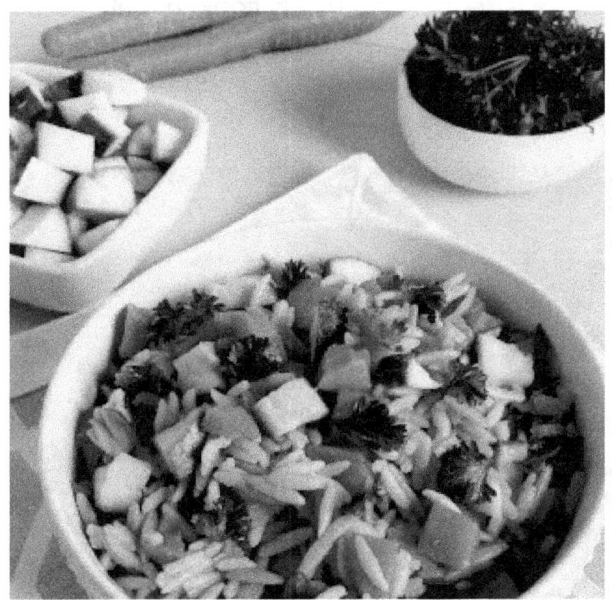

Image: www.yummly.com

Ingredients:

1/3 cup basmati rice
¼ tsp black pepper
2 whole carrot
¼ inch fresh ginger
½ whole lime
¼ tsp mineral salt
1 tbsp sunflower oil
4 cups of water
1 cup of Zucchini

Instructions:

Boil the water. Dice the Zucchini and the carrots and grate the ginger. Mix everything with water and bring to a boil. Reduce the heat and simmer.

Wait till the rice is tender and nicely cooked. Eat when hot.

Curried Chick Pea with Carrots

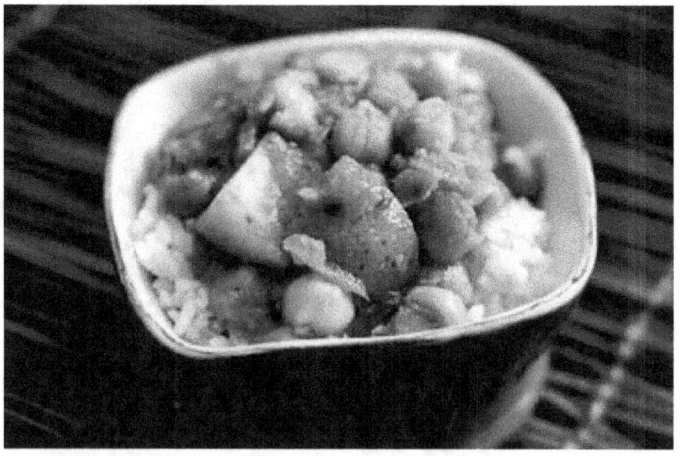

Source: www.simplyrecipes.com

Ingredients:

½ tsp of black salt
6 carrots
¼ tsp cayenne pepper
1 cup chick pea
¼ tsp cinnamon
½ tsp cloves
½ tsp cumin
¼ tsp fenugreek
½ tsp ginger
1 tbsp olive oil
2 tomatoes
1/3 cup yellow onion

Instructions:

Grind well and mix all the spices to form a paste. Chop the tomatoes and crush them well. Sate the onions and the other spices in oil and stir well.

After the onions are brown, add the other ingredients and a little water. Cover it. Reduce the heat and bring it to a boil.

Wait till the carrots are tender. Mix well and serve/eat hot.

Ayurvedic Dinner Recipes

Holiday Spice Blend – Churna

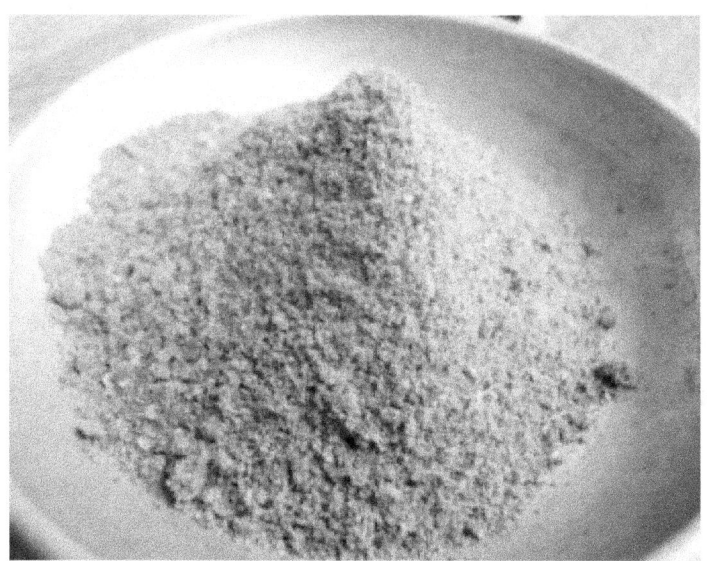

Source: www.etsy.com

Ingredients:
1 tsp cardamom
1 tbsp cinnamon
1 tsp cloves
2 tbsp coriander seeds
1 tbsp cumin
2 tsp fennel seeds
1 tbsp dried ginger
½ tsp mineral salt
1 tbsp Sucanat
1 tbsp turmeric

Instructions:

Add all the ingredients and dry blend them. Once the powder is obtained, it can be used with any meal.

Churna can be added to all soups, and almost all Ayurvedic foods. The soups and broth recipes will follow. Store the churna in an air-tight container and use whenever required.

Yoghurt & Cumin Digestive Lassi

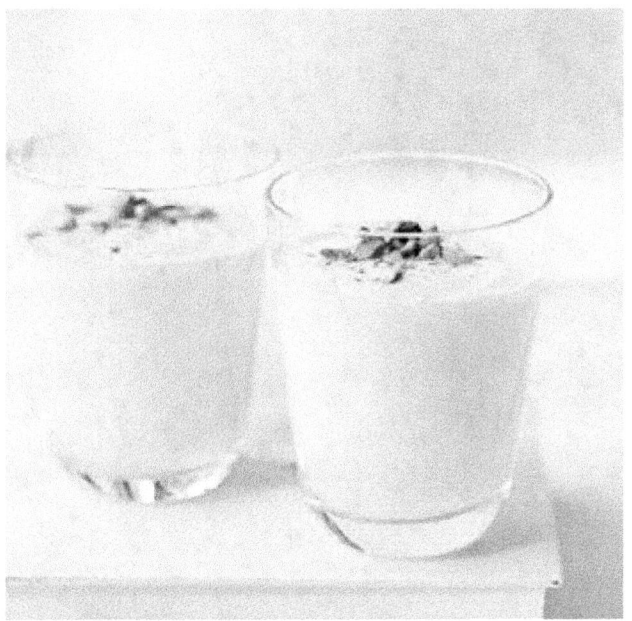

Source: wandernosh.com

Ingredients:

¼ tsp Cumin
1 lemon wedge
2 pinches of salt
2/3 cups of water
1/3 cups yoghurt

Instructions:

Put all the ingredients in a blender and blend until smooth. Can be served directly or chilled, and later served.

However, it tastes best when chilled.

Buttery Carrot Soup

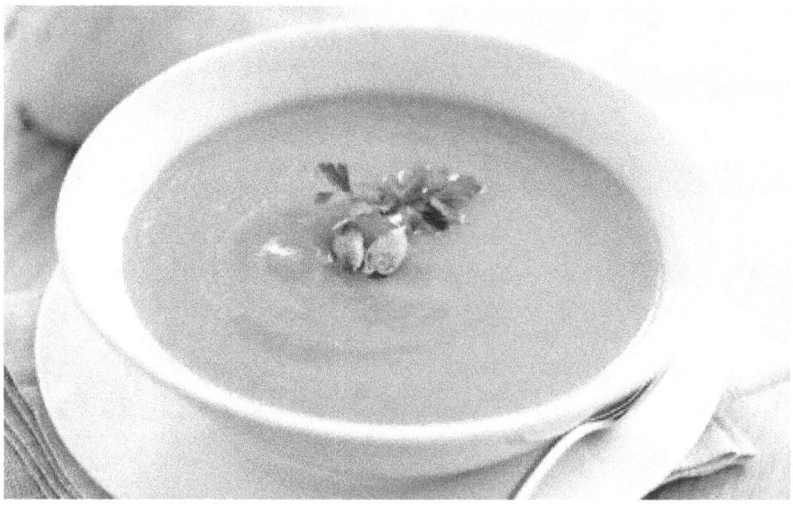

Source: www.andreabeaman.com

Ingredients:

1 Bay leaf
2 pinches black pepper
2 tbsp butter
4 whole carrots
1 clove of garlic
¼ tsp mineral salt
1 tsp fresh thyme
4 cups of water

¼ cups yellow onion

Instructions:

Saute onions in the butter along with garlic until the onions turn golden brown. Blend the onions and the carrot in the blender. Add some water and then pulse them slightly.

Pour the contents of the blender into the pot and boil for 15 minutes. Serve hot.

Beet Cleanse Soup

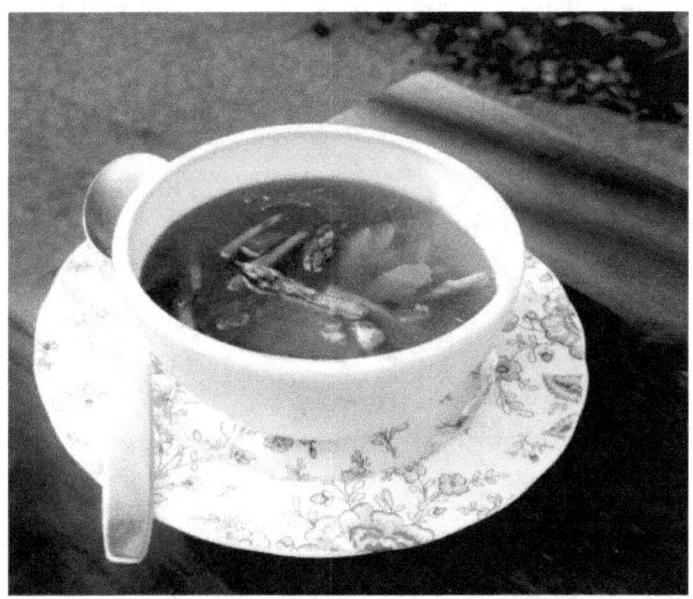

Image: honestfare.com

Ingredients:

3 tbsp Apple Cider vinegar
2 cups diced beetroot
¼ tsp black pepper

2 cups cooked cabbage
4 carrots
3/4 cups dill
1 potato
¼ tsp mineral salt
2 tbsp sunflower oil
½ cups yellow onion

Instructions:

Chop the onions, potatoes, carrots, beets and cabbages. Put all the ingredients in a pot and cover well.

Heat up the pot well, bring it to a boil and simmer. Cover it for one hour.

Add the churna, or garlic and parsley as extra ingredients.

Sweet Turnips with Ghee

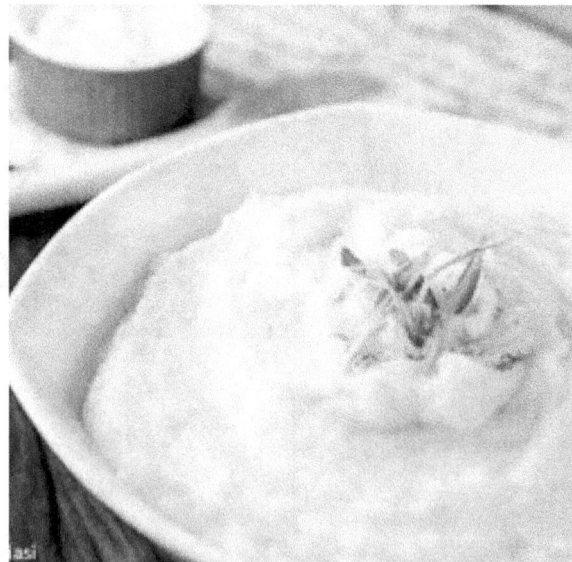

Source: www.joyfulbelly.com

Ingredients:
1 tbsp ghee
¼ tsp salt
4 cups turnip

Instructions:

Peel the turnips, wash them well, and rinse for some time. After a few minutes, chop them and set aside,.

Boil water in a pot and add all the ingredients. Reduce the flames or bring to a simmer and allow to cook for one hour. Stir occasionally.

After an hour, mash the contents of the pot, or pulse with a blender.

Cabbage Soup Diet

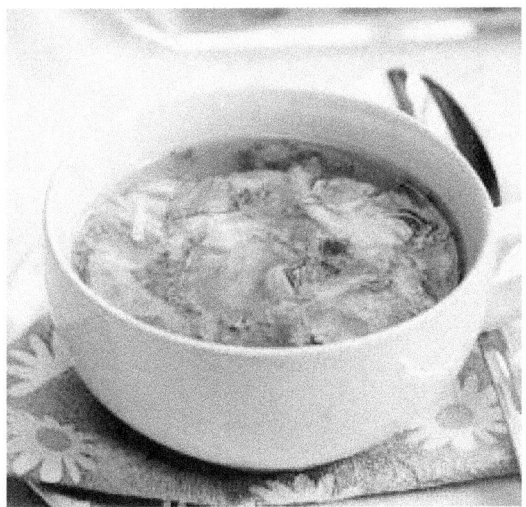

Source: dietliedel.atspace.co.uk

Ingredients:

¼ tsp black pepper
4 cups cooked cabbage
½ tsp mineral salt
¼ cups yellow onion
¼ cups celery stalk
¼ tsp curry or churna powder
1 garlic clove
¼ cup Fresh Parsley

Instructions:

Add all the ingredients in a pot. Pour water to cover the vegetables, bring to a boil, and simmer.

Allow all the ingredients to cook for 45 to 50 minutes. Stir occasionally. When the vegetables are tender, you can remove them from the stove and serve.

A Small Recap - Happy Detox!

Ayurveda is one of the world's oldest medicinal practices. As mentioned in many places in this book, Ayurveda is completely natural, and the way you will detox your body is all the same. There are many claims stating that Ayurveda Detox is just a myth, but as far as we know, it works.

If you had read this book, we are sure you will have an idea that it works too. Ayurveda also has many scientific explanations. Though these are ancient practices, they are still very effective in the modern world.

More than 90% of the people who go through Ayurvedic detox have found it to be effective. We hope that you could be one of them too. If you follow all the instructions given in this book, you will surely find it to be effective.

In case you have been reading this book for too long, then here is a quick recap of what you have read.

1. Find your Dosha

Your Dosha is the key to detox. Find out which your body type is and choose the Doshas accordingly. Once you determine your dosha, you will have to optimize your diet accordingly.

2. Undergo all the Three Stages

Strictly follow the pre detox, detox and post detox stages. These are very essential. DO not skip any stage, because all of them are equally important. Ayurvedic Detox takes time, but the more Slowly you do it, the more effective it will be.

3. Be Consistent

Be consistent in whatever you do. Do not go too slow or too fast during the detox process. For any process, consistency is the key. Ayurveda is no different. Since Ayurveda is a natural treatment, it normally takes longer than the other artificial ones.

4. Take care of digestion

The digestive system has to perform properly. Eat lots of ghee and selected oils during the stages.

5. Cleanliness

Maintain cleanliness and hygiene throughout the detoxification process. Toxifying your body while detoxifying it will prove the whole detoxification process useless.

6. Always Ask for Expert Help

If you find anything abnormal during your detox process, always make sure that you consult a physician, preferably an Ayurveda expert.

We wish you all the best for your detox. It is not a very difficult task, at least not that difficult when compared to climbing Mount Everest. There are testimonials of many people who have experienced the positive effects of Ayurvedic detoxification. You can find them on the internet.

Above all, believe in yourself. Self confidence is one of the best friends of Ayurvedic treatment. If you are confident about what you are doing, then you will surely be able to achieve the desired results.

Try not to give up once you start the detox process. Of course, in dire situations, you will have no other option, but try to get yourself together and go through it. There might be many problems that might come and go, but set yourself on your goal, focus it, and carry on.

Once you finish the detox process successfully, you can still stick to the Ayurvedic way of life. Many people who have tried this have become so accustomed to the process, that they have made it their lifestyle. You could very well be one of them too. Always remember that Ayurveda has no side effects or complications.

So get your body, mind and soul prepared and start the detox process. Happy detox!

Don't forget ! Get your Free report giveaway here
http://wellnesshealthhub.com/ayurvedic-report

Find out more about the author: **Monica Ramirez**

Website: www.wellnesshealthhub.com